Binge Eating

How to End Emotional Eating and Start a Successful Weight Loss

By: Crystal Stevens

Introduction

This book contains proven steps and strategies on how to finally stop the unhealthy eating habit known as binge eating. Medically considered as a disorder, binge eating has many negative effects on your mental, emotional, and physical health. You may not be aware of it now, but you will surely regret it in the future — when you're already trapped in this vicious and unhealthy cycle.

Stress, anxiety, depression and other unhealthy emotions can really get the best of us, and we sometimes tend to deal with them through comfort eating. While indulging in your favorite meals and snacks once in a while is not bad, overeating at frequent periods of time and more than what you can handle is obviously detrimental to your well-being.

This book will show you that overeating is not the answer to your problems. Whether you have a serious weight issue or you're trying to battle depression, stuffing your mouth with unhealthy choices of food will not improve your situation. Yes, it might temporarily lighten up your mood, but the long-term effect is not always favorable.

Are you ready to destroy your binge eating behavior and start a successful weight loss plan instead? Continue to read this book and you will definitely gems of information to help you improve your life, health, and overall well-being

I hope you enjoy it!

Chapter 1: What is Binge Eating?

Did you ever find yourself in a situation wherein you feel unable to control yourself from eating too much during a small period of time, like two to three hours of uncontrollable overeating?

Not to be confused with occasional situations like having more than a few servings during a holiday dinner party or going over the top when in an all-you-can-eat restaurant, or when stuffing yourself to the point of throwing up when trying to win an eating contest, the uncontrollable overeating episodes I was referring to seem to occur randomly and almost regularly up to almost a few times each week.

These episodes can be referred to as binge eating episodes and can be very harmful to your health if it gets out of hand.

Binge eating episodes are often triggered by some distressing emotions and may be a behavioral manifestation of a deeper affective and psychological issue, especially if it is a persistent occurrence. If these episodes occur regularly and an overwhelming feeling of regret, shame, and guilt comes to you right after your episodes, and these episodes start to affect your daily activities and your health, it is imperative that you get yourself diagnosed if you are suffering from binge eating disorder.

Let's look at what this disorder actually is in more detail to give you a better understanding of what you may be going through.

You probably picked this book because episodes like the one mentioned above is familiar to you and you are figuring out if you have the disorder or not. Maybe it isn't you who have experienced these episodes, but you suspect a loved one to be having difficulty controlling their eating behavior and you are concerned.

The fact that you are reading this means that you have acknowledged the problem and you are ready to work on yourself or others in order to correct this harmful eating behavior. Read on to find out if you or your loved one have the disorder or may be on the way to developing such condition.

What is Binge Eating Disorder?

Binge eating disorder has been recently added to the Diagnostic and Statistical Manual of Mental Disorders, 5th edition, indicating that it is now a disorder on its own, as opposed to it being formerly categorized as a sub-type of EDNOS or eating disorders otherwise not specified.

Binge eating disorder is diagnosed by the occurrence of the following criteria:

- Persistent episodes of binge eating. Episodes are characterized by a feeling of being unable to stop eating at a certain period and consuming more than the normal amount of food for a short period of time.

- Binge eating episodes are identified if it occurs alongside at least three of the following:

  - Eating faster than normal

  - Sensation of being too full

  - Lack of physical hunger sensation yet eating more than usual

  - Feeling the need to hide the eating episode from others because of shame

  - Guilt, embarrassment, or disgust after each episode

- Emotional distress associated with binge eating

- Frequent and persistent occurrence of episodes, with at least one episode per week lasting for at least three months

It is important also to note that binge eating episodes that characterize the disorder should occur independently of other eating disorders such as the purging episodes associated with bulimia nervosa. Purging that sometimes occur after a binge eating episode is a behavioral manifestation of the guilt and regret that one feels for consuming too much food, and it is independent of bulimia which is a different eating disorder.

Symptoms and Warnings Signs: Do You Have Binge Eating Disorder?

It is possible that you or your loved one is not diagnosed with the disorder, yet you experience binge eating episodes frequently that causes negative effects on the mental and physical state.

Some of the warning signs that you need to be wary of are the following because you or your loved one may be on the way to developing the full-fledged disorder and it is imperative to stop the behaviors before it gets worse.

1. If it is not yourself that is suffering from the eating disorder, you should be wary of evidences of binge eating in your household, such as finding food or snack wrappers in the bin, losing a large amount of food for a short period of time, or anything else that indicates over consumption of food.

2. Feeling uneasy or being fearful when eating with other people, as people who binge would rather eat alone due to the feeling of being judged negatively for their poor food choices.

3. People who binge eat are always ready to try new fad diets and extreme diets, such as extremely low calorie count diet to compensate for the overeating.

4. Food hoarding

5. Canceling plans or scheduling one's weekly activities to make time for binge eating episodes

6. Avoiding friends and usual activities

7. Always dieting and trying new ways to lose weight

8. Being overcritical about own body shape and flaws

9. Abnormal eating behaviors such as unusual amount of food, irregular eating time, and skipping meals that indicate disruption in daily eating habits

10. Extreme and fast weight changes

11. Stomach disorders such as acid reflux, indigestion, constipation or abdominal cramps

12. Inability to focus

There are other warning signs that may make a person more prone to developing binge eating disorder such as low self-esteem, high expectations about one's own physical appearance, high concern for other people's opinion of oneself, and body dissatisfaction.

What Causes People to Binge?

There are social, physiological, and psychological factors that influence people to engage in binge eating behaviors that may eventually lead to binge eating disorder.

Some of the social risk factors that increase the likelihood of developing binge eating disorder include the following.

1. Societal beauty standards

The various forms of media, especially social media, have been shaping the beauty standards of people in most places in the world. Because of these, people perceive being overweight as unattractive, and skinny as attractive.

Runway models, magazine cover girls, television and movie celebrities, pop stars, social media influencers, and other personalities that people look up to propagate the stigma that being fat is not desirable. This stigma is a large influence on how people behave in terms of eating habits and other fitness practices.

2. Weight shaming

People who develop eating disorders, specifically binge eating behaviors, are likely to have been bullied or teased because of their weight. In most social circles, including schools or the workplace, insensitivity to weight issues has been very common. Whether it is a blatant bullying attack on someone's weight or a subtle joke about being fat, these social situations often lead someone to develop unusual dieting habits to ward of the ridicule or shame that they experience.

3. Westernization

Even in places where beauty standards on body size were varied, the relatively recent Westernization of foreign nations have contributed a lot to the prevalence of eating disorders and binge eating behaviors. For instance, countries where fuller body shapes have been celebrated over the years have recently been seen to conform to western body images and standards, due to the introduction of Western influences through art, media, and social media, people who engage in eating behaviors that result in drastic weight changes have increased.

4. Lack of socialization

Studies have shown that being lonely or not having friends is correlated to binge eating behaviors. The lack of social support and positive social interactions and activities may cause a person who is already having some body issues to spin into uncontrollable and harmful eating habits to feel better about themselves.

The development of binge eating disorder is a combination of factors. There is not one single cause or event that triggers a person to start binge eating. However, there are some psychological factors that make a person more prone to developing binge eating disorder and behaviors. Some of these psychological factors include:

1. Being too self-critical

Eating disorders have been shown to be related to perfectionism and being over critical about ones' self. The link between perfectionism and binge eating is related to having elevated standards about yourself that you tend to do push yourself even to the point of hurting yourself just to achieve your unrealistically high standards

2. Ideal body dissonance

Related to perfectionism, having a psychological issue about how your actual body does not fit your ideal body may also trigger you to develop binge eating behaviors. If you feel that you are too fat or too skinny as compared to the ideal body size that you have in your head, you might be psychologically prone to engaging in harmful eating patterns.

3. Body dismorphia

This is a type of disorder where you over magnify your own physical flaws. It is a psychological condition wherein you make your negative physical attributes more noticeable than they really are to outsider's perspective. People with this type of disorder tend to do drastic and often harmful procedures to correct these real or imagined flaws.

A person with body dismorphia may see himself or herself as obese when in reality, they are underweight. So they continue with their harmful eating habits just to lose the imaginary weight.

4. Anxiety disorder

Having some form of an anxiety disorder has been linked to eating disorders. The disorders may be comorbid, suggesting that some underlying factor caused both disorders or one may have caused the other. It is reasonable to believe that people who have anxiety disorder may be too worried about things and feel that they cannot control anything, that they tend to engage in harmful practices that might make the anxiety ebb. Thus, someone who has social anxiety may engage in binge eating behaviors to be liked by others; or someone with obsessive compulsive disorder may binge eat because of one's compulsion to food.

5. Lack of behavioral adjustment

People who have eating disorders, including those who binge eat have a higher tendency to be a person who follows rules, and does everything with the right order and procedure. These people who are unable to bend their own rules are likely to be too conscious about what their own habits, but may lose control when eating. They gain control back by forcing themselves to get sick and avoid the consequences of eating too much.

Some people may also be genetically predisposed to having eating disorders. People with relatives who have anxiety disorders or eating disorders have a higher likelihood of developing an eating disorder, suggesting that there might be a gene that increases the proneness to maladaptive eating patterns.

Furthermore, people who have genetically low metabolism rate have also been reported to have a higher tendency to binge eat. The combination of the genetic, social. and psychological factors all contribute to the development of an eating disorder that may push a person to repeatedly engage in harmful eating behaviors such as binge eating.

How Emotions Affect People's Eating Habits and Behaviors

Have you ever experienced eating too much junk food like chips, fast food, chocolates, and ice cream after a break up, or after getting fired from work, or failing a class in school? These instances happen because you may have used food as your coping mechanism whenever something bad happens to you.

Binge eating episodes are often triggered by an external event that causes an emotional reaction, which then triggers the person to seek comfort in food.

Most people find comfort in eating but, it is often a temporary fix to a long-term emotional distress. Thus, you become trapped in a vicious cycle of overeating, because your emotional hunger cannot be satiated. Furthermore, the more you overeat to compensate for your negative emotions, the worse you will feel after, because of all the weight you are putting on. As a result, you may feel sadder about your physical appearance or you get more situations that make you feel down such as being ridiculed for your weight. Then the cycle starts all over again. This is why binge eating behaviors can lead to binge eating disorder wherein the episodes happen regularly.

For some people who binge eat, it is not only sadness or anxiety that triggers an episode. Any form of stress, anger, tiredness, or even just boredom can push someone to a binge eating episode. This is why it is important to understand what you are feeling — whether it is emotional hunger or actual physiological hunger. The former cannot be satiated by eating food. Thus you may be better off dealing with your emotions directly and not try to escape by using food.

Why Binge Eating is Unhealthy and Why You Need to End it Now

You may feel good momentarily while you are throwing down that milkshake and scarfing down those potato chips, but that feeling of escape, comfort, and satisfaction will soon end, and you will be left with nothing but guilt, shame, embarrassment, and regret shortly after. You may also develop some anxiety and depression due to your inability to face your emotions and lack of control of your own behavior.

In addition, you will have an overall lower quality of life due to the isolation that you put yourself into. Most people who binge eat hide the evidences and symptoms of the disorder from their friends and loved ones, causing the feeling of loneliness and isolation.

Not only is binge eating negative for your mental health, your physical health will also suffer from this practice. For one thing, you will definitely gain weight from binge eating, even if you try to force yourself to get sick and throw up. Chances are, your body will crave to replace the lost fuel, so it is probable that your episodes of binge eating will only increase and become more frequent as opposed to when you do not throw up all the food you consumed.

So, apart from being depressed, lonely, ashamed, and guilty, you will also be fat and unhealthy because of this behavior. You will also most likely suffer stomach cramps and other digestive problems. You should also be wary of other diseases associated with obesity and overeating such as diabetes, high blood pressure, cardiovascular diseases, gallbladder problems, and cholesterol issues.

If you are experiencing emotions-triggered overeating and bouts of binge eating, it is imperative that you stop the behavior right now before it spirals out of control. The following chapter will help you fight against the impulse and make better eating decisions. If you think that you are suffering from binge eating disorder as described above, it is recommended that you seek medical and professional advice immediately.

* * * * *

CHAPTER SUMMARY:

- Binge eating disorder is often characterized by a feeling of being unable to stop eating, consuming more than the normal amount of food for a short period of time, and then being guilty, embarrassed, or disgusted after each episode.

- It is important to identify early warning signs of binge eating disorder in order to take proper actions. Some symptoms include food hoarding, trying new fad diets and extreme diets, being overcritical about weight and figure, abnormal eating behaviors, fast weight changes, and stomach disorders.

- There are a couple of social, physiological, and psychological factors that influence people to engage in binge eating behaviors.

- Binge eating episodes are often triggered by an external event that causes an emotional reaction, such as anxiety, stress, or even boredom.

- Binge eating brings many negative effects on your physical and mental health. It is imperative that you stop the behavior now before it spirals out of control.

Chapter 2: Proven Ways to Stop Binge Eating

If you have been battling with episodes of binge eating, here are some ways that will help you win over negative eating habits and become healthier.

1. Eat regularly.

Studies have shown that eating well-balanced meal at regular intervals decreases the frequency of binge eating. Try setting a schedule of when you will eat and make sure to stick to it as much as you can.

Skipping a meal will only lead to higher levels of blood sugar and will trigger the production of hunger stimulating hormone called ghrelin. The higher level of this hormone in your body, the higher the likelihood that you will have cravings. If you get cravings, for a person who binge eats, this may mean another episode of binge eating that will leave you guilty and regretful.

2. Don't restrict yourself.

Most fad diets involve restricting yourself from consuming one food group and loading up on another. Totally restricting your diet will only lead to cravings that are hard to ignore. So for instance, going on a low-carb diet and restricting yourself from eating anything sugary will only lead you to crave foods that are high in sugar. This craving will persist until you give in.

Thus, if you are already battling binge eating behavior, putting yourself on a diet will only put you in a path wherein your will power will be constantly tested. And once you give in to your cravings, a binge eating cycle may ensue.

Furthermore, fasting and cutting calories have also been shown to increase the tendency of over eating in most women.

Thus, it is better to just stick to a schedule of eating, and eat a well-balanced diet with controlled portions.

3. Practice mindful eating.

Now that you already know the difference between psychical hunger and hunger triggered by your emotions, you will be better able to react to your triggers. By being mindful of your mind and body, you can easily avoid emotional eating. You can do this by listening to your body. Ask yourself if you are really hungry or maybe your emotions are just driving you to eat more.

If you are already eating, be in the moment. Do not just scarf down everything in front of you. Enjoy the moment and savor every bite of food you consume. By doing this, you become more aware of your satiation and hence, you stop eating once you are full.

4. Drink more water.

Drinking water helps you feel fuller and thus, decreasing the likelihood of feeling hungry. So drink water regularly throughout the day and keep those cravings at bay.

Water has been proven to help decrease calorie intake by taking up the space in your stomach that will otherwise be occupied by food. Thus, if you want to eat less, try drinking water before your meals. And if you find yourself in an uncontrollable binge eating episode, try drinking water instead.

However, you should still keep in mind that drinking too much might be bad for you in some case, as some bodies require more hydration than others. This is where mindfulness becomes helpful. Listen to your body and drink when you are thirsty. But drinking 8 glasses of water per day or up to 2 liters of water is never bad for any body type.

5. Try anxiety-reducing activities.

If you are an emotional eater and you tend to stuff your face when you are feeling stressed, you should probably try some alternative activities. You know yourself pretty well, so you should know what can help you reduce the stress that you are feeling other than overeating. For instance, instead of reaching for the refrigerator and devouring everything in it after a stressful day at work, try doing something else that calms you down. Maybe take up a new hobby, like painting, gardening, or reading.

One way to calm your emotions and be more mindful of what your body wants and needs, is to do some yoga. Yoga makes you become more aware of your breathing and the sensations of your body, making you feel more relaxed. It has been proven to reduce cortisol, the stress hormone, and decreases the chances of body dissatisfaction and depression.

6. Stock up on healthy food.

Binge eating episodes usually only happens at home, away from the eyes of others who may judge you negatively. Almost always when something triggers your overeating tendencies, you will reach for the nearest junk food and start from there. If your kitchen or pantry does not have any of those processed junk food and sugary foods, then there is nothing to binge on.

Alternatively, if you stock up your pantry with fruits and vegetables, whole grains, nuts and protein foods, you will be more equipped to make better healthy choices when your food cravings come rolling in.

7. Eat a high-protein and high-fiber breakfast.

Breakfast is the most important meal of the day. It fuels you up for the morning and most of the day. Skipping breakfast will only lead you to being sluggish throughout the day, feeling hungry, and having cravings. It is a good idea to stock up on protein and fiber in the morning to reduce the production of ghrelin, the hunger hormone, throughout the day.

Furthermore, eating breakfast helps you feel fuller longer throughout he day, eliminating the need for snacking. It will help you curb your appetite and avoid overeating.

8. Increase physical activities.

Whenever you feel stressed, sad, or any other emotion that triggers your binge eating behavior, go out and do some running or brisk walking to calm you down and relax you. Physical activities and exercise have been proven to reduce anxiety and decease the probability of over eating. So when you feel the urge to binge, distract yourself by engaging in physical activities.

Join a gym and start a regular exercise routine. Not only will this make you look and feel better and help with your body satisfaction, this will also assist in focusing on your body and developing the awareness on what your body needs.

9. Get quality sleep.

Sleeping eight hours per day have been shown to greatly reduce binge-eating behavior. Sleep also helps curb your appetite and reduces hunger throughout the day.

People who do not get enough quality sleep have reported to have higher binge eating tendencies and higher levels of ghrelin in their body. Furthermore, lack of sleep increases stress levels even when doing simple tasks, which might lead you to overeat.

10. Eat more protein.

Protein in your diet increases the feeling of fullness, decreasing your tendency to overeat. According to a study, eating a high protein breakfast will decrease your appetite longer, keeping you feeling full the whole morning as it increases the production of hormones that controls appetite. It also reduces the amount of calories you ingest during lunch.

Protein also helps in boosting your metabolism and aids in fat loss. Twenty to 30 per cent of your caloric intake is recommended to come from protein. In order to achieve this, always incorporate high-protein food source in every meal. Eggs are packed with healthy fats and high amount of protein, which makes you feel full longer. Other sources of protein include salmon, tuna, almonds, milk, broccoli, Greek yogurt, spinach, lean beef, chicken breasts and other red meat, and seafood.

11. Follow a meal plan.

Make sure to plan your healthy meals for the whole week. This will help you keep healthy ingredients in your kitchen that will allow you to whip up a nutritious meal when you need it.

A meal plan will help you stick to your schedule and will keep you from overeating on junk and processed foods. Advanced meal planning has been shown to reduce the risk of obesity and binge eating, and increases the quality and variety of meals.

12. Keep track of your meals and your moods.

Keeping a food journal is known to reduce calorie intake and increased long-term weight management. A journal will also help you adhere to your diet, making it less likely for you to binge on high-calorie snacks.

In addition, it is a good idea to track your moods and emotions to increase your awareness of what triggers your binge eating episodes. Knowing your triggers will help you to better avoid them. Furthermore, it puts more responsibility on yourself to make better food choices and improve your eating habits.

13. Find a support group.

Since loneliness and depression have been identified as correlates of binge eating disorder, and negative emotions from being alone and isolated may trigger binge eating, it is a good idea to seek a friend and start talking to someone whenever you feel the urge to binge. If you are not comfortable yet to talk about your eating problems, you can always talk about anything else, as long as it distracts you from the emotions that trigger your binge eating episodes.

It is also better for your mental health to find other people who have similar struggles as you do in terms of why you are binge eating. They may offer more insight and better advice on how to stop, and they can help you realize things about yourself that you formerly could not see from your own perspective.

Your support group can help you figure out what causes you to binge, what exactly your triggers are, and how you can fight against your compulsions.

If all the other strategies that were presented to you have failed in stopping you from binge eating, then it is time for you to admit to yourself that the problem is much bigger than yourself and you need to involve other people in your path to recovery. Seek professional help when you feel the behavior is getting out of control and you cannot fight it on your own.

* * * * *

CHAPTER SUMMARY:

- There are effective ways on how to stop or minimize binge eating episodes. These include eating regularly and at a scheduled time, practicing mindful eating, stocking up on healthy food, and following a meal plan.

- Specific foods and drinks that will help you manage your condition includes water, high-protein meals, and high-fiber foods.

- Furthermore, lifestyle changes like increasing physical activities, getting enough sleep, and finding a support group.

- Seek professional help when you feel the behavior is getting out of control and you cannot fight it on your own.

Chapter 3: Healthier Alternatives to Weight Loss

Although fad diets almost never work, especially for a person who is not committed to doing it in the long-term, there are diets that you can try to help curb your cravings and reduce the likelihood of a binge-eating episode.

The key to choosing the right diet for a person who has an eating disorder, binge eating to be exact, is to provide yourself with ample nutrition and small indulgences which will stop you from having cravings and from overindulging on certain times. It is also important to be consistent with whatever meal plan you choose to use.

Here are some dieting alternatives that you can try that have been evaluated to be safe and effective for those who want to lose weight but have the tendency to over-indulge.

Low-Carb Diets

There are several low-carb diets that people use for weight loss, but they all have the same idea. The key is to limit the amount of carbohydrates in your diet to only 20 to 150 grams daily, while giving you the freedom to consume protein and fat without restrictions. The idea is to keep the body from using carbs as its fuel source, rather the body will use up the fatty acids that will be transformed as ketones that the body can use as energy. This process burns fat and assists in weight loss.

Low-carb diets reduce your appetite, and have been shown by several studies to be very effective in helping obese and overweight people lose weight. The aim of low-carb diets is to reach ketosis, or the burning of fat to create ketones for the body to use as energy. This is the principle behind the Keto diet which involves the consumption of fats instead of carbs. Ketosis can also be achieved through intermittent fasting, which involves not eating anything for at least 16 hours per day, and having no limitations as to what you will eat in the remaining 8-hour feeding window.

For low-carb diet, keto diet, and intermittent fasting, the effectiveness and the suitability vary for each person. It is important to consult a medical practitioner to help you figure out if the diet is suitable for you, after considering your medical history and current health condition.

However, intermittent fasting is not recommended for people who have e tendency to binge eat. Keeping yourself from eating for a long period of time will only escalate your cravings and will lead to binge eating during the feeding windows which will result to weight gain if you cannot manage the amount of food you eat during the said amount of time.

Keto diet may also be problematic for people who have the urge to binge, as it limits their food intake and does not allow them to have tiny indulgences on carbs and sweets, thus increasing the likelihood of a binge relapse.

The low-carb diet may be a good weight loss diet alternative that will help you curb your appetite as eating more proteins will keep you fuller for longer and it will allow you to have your little indulgences as long as you restrict the amount that you eat.

Low-Fat Diets

Low-fat diets typically recommend consumption of less than 30% calories from fat, and ultra low fat diets restrict fat calories to less than 15%. The idea behind the fat restriction is that a gram of fat contains more calories as compared to a gram of protein or carbs. Thus, you consume fewer calories for more food intake if you limit the calories from fat.

Low-fat diet has been shown to help in improving blood pressure and other cardiovascular diseases. It also helps in fighting type II diabetes. Its effectiveness in weight loss has been seen to be significant for those who are obese and overweight. However, recent studies have shown that ultra low fat diets are less effective in weigh loss as compared to the low-carb diet.

The difficulty with low-fat diet for people who have the tendency to binge eat is that it may seem unsustainable due to the lack of variety. It is also often not satisfying in terms of taste, and as a result, some people may tend to relapse while on this diet.

Low-Calorie Diets

The idea behind the low-calorie diet is that you can continue to eat what you normally eat without restricting any food group, but with controlled portions to restrict the amount of calories ingested. For instance, you normally consume 2000 calories per day from all sources of calories such as protein, fats, and carbs; a low-calorie diet will have you eating 1700 calories of the same food. This may also suggest opting to eat a healthier alternative to your normal food which has fewer calories.

This type of diet may be helpful for a person who is trying to stop binge eating. The key to the effectiveness of this weight loss strategy is consistency and careful tracking. This is where your mood and food journal may come in handy. You can keep track of the calories you have had in the day by calculating the calories in all the food you had that day.

This diet does not restrict you from your little indulgences that helps reduce cravings, and it allows you to plan your meals throughout the day with little adjustments to portion sizes.

However, just like all other diets, it is important to seek medical advice before starting as most diets are not for everyone.

* * * * *

CHAPTER SUMMARY:

- If you are trying to lose weight, but your binge eating disorder prevents you from successfully achieving it, there are healthier diet alternatives you may consider.

- Low-carb diets reduce your appetite, and have been shown by several studies to be very effective in helping obese and overweight people lose weight.

- Low-fat diets typically recommend consumption of less than 30% calories from fat, and ultra low fat diets restrict fat calories to less than 15%.

- The idea behind the low-calorie diet is that you can continue to eat what you normally eat without restricting any food group, but with controlled portions to restrict the amount of calories ingested.

Chapter 4: Managing Your Emotions and Making Lifestyles Changes

If you have tried altering your diet and your daily eating habits, but still find yourself relapsing ad having binge eating episodes, do not panic and do not lose heart. Maybe it is time to make a commitment to a lifestyle change that you can stick to. This chapter will help you deal with relapses and making long-term changes to completely stop binge eating.

Here are some things to remember when completely changing your lifestyle to prevent yourself from relapsing into another binge eating episode

1. Be committed and be consistent.

Changing your lifestyle does not happen overnight. It will probably take you weeks, months, or even years to completely remove overeating in your system. As it was established earlier, binge eating is a cycle of environmental stressors and emotional triggers that repeats itself over again due to the stress that overeating and weight gain has on a person prone to body dissatisfaction.

So keep in mind that stopping this cycle will require hard work. It is not easy, but it is doable, if you fully commit to changing your habits. The changes do not stop once you achieve a goal weight or body; it is a continuous effort in order to beat the cycle.

2. Be observant about yourself.

Part of being constantly mindful is to observe your body and your mind. You should know the signs when you are starting to slip into binge eating again. If you are constantly feeling anxious or nervous, if you are feeling embarrassed or ashamed about eating, if you are becoming more of a loner, if you are being more critical about the way you look, you may be starting to relapse again. So try to do the strategies above in order to help you distract yourself from eating.

Part of being observant is also knowing what your triggers are. If you know you tend to overindulge if you get stressed by your boss or by your kids, then you would know how to avoid these kinds of stress. So the next time your boss gives you a hard time, stop and meditate before getting yourself too stressed out that you start binge eating again. Maybe blow off some steam by hitting the gym or going for a run.

3. Don't be too hard on yourself.

You may have stopped binge eating for about three months and you suddenly find yourself in another uncontrollable eating episode when a sudden unexpected event stressed you out. Don't put yourself down about one relapse, it happens occasionally to most people. What you should be focusing on is how you can immediately go back to your regular schedule and eating patterns.

Set a plan that will put you back on track and do not go full-on relapse as you wight get sucked into the binge eating cycle again.

It also does not help if you are too strict about your diet. You are allowed to indulge on the things that make you happy. Just make sure to control how much you eat. So the next time you have a hankering for some chocolate ice cream, allow yourself to have half a cup. Just don't get a whole tub and keep it in your fridge, as this will only tempt you to break your diet.

4. Add variety to your days.

Being bored with the routine of your days can trigger overeating and may cause you to be more stressed than usual. So treat yourself occasionally, maybe go out on a holiday, and de-stress from work. Instead of going on the same way to do your errands, maybe take a different route. Who knows what you may discover along the way? Instead of eating at home alone, try eating out with your friends. The next time you get a craving of something, try eating it outside or with the company of other people to prevent you from over indulging.

5. Learn to distract yourself.

Emotional eating is always triggered by how you feel at the moment. If you can distract yourself from what you are feeling long enough for you to calm yourself down and think more clearly, you can avoid relapsing every time you get stressed. So if you are feeling the urge to overeat, try to relax and meditate. If that is not your kind of thing, maybe try another activity, or better yet, invite some friends over to help you feel good about yourself.

6. Practice positive self-talk.

Learn to appreciate yourself for who you are. Instead of focusing on what you don't like abut your body, try looking at yourself in a more positive light. Focus on what makes you beautiful, even if you do not have the body of a supermodel or a social media fitness influencer. You have your own specific qualities that make you a beautiful person inside and out. So next time you look in the mirror, instead of looking at your flaws with a magnifying glass, try to tell yourself how amazing you are. This will not only make you feel good about your body image, but it will also take all the pressure of being perfect away from your mind.

Positive self-talk also helps in your path to stopping binge eating altogether. Whenever you have a stressful day or you feel sad, talk to yourself in a positive manner. Tell yourself that you are confident and strong, and you can get through any adversity without having to resort to harmful habits that will only set you back. Whenever you are starting to relapse, you can tell yourself you can get back up again and set yourself on track. This way, nothing will ever get you down.

* * * * *

CHAPTER SUMMARY:

- To fully be successful at putting an end to your binge eating episodes and maintain a healthy living, you need to learn how to manage your emotions and make some permanent lifestyle changes.

- These include being committed and consistent, being observant about yourself, adding variety to your days, and practicing positive self talk.

Conclusion

I hope this book was able to help you learn more about binge eating disorder and how serious it can affect your mental, emotional, and physical health.

The next step is to take action and overcome this unhealthy eating habit. It may take a lot of work, commitment, and perseverance, but remember that you are doing this for yourself and not for anyone. Binge eating is an unpleasant cycle that you don't want to be trapped in. So, before it gets out of control, start making small changes to your daily eating habits and lifestyle and successfully end the binge eating disorder.

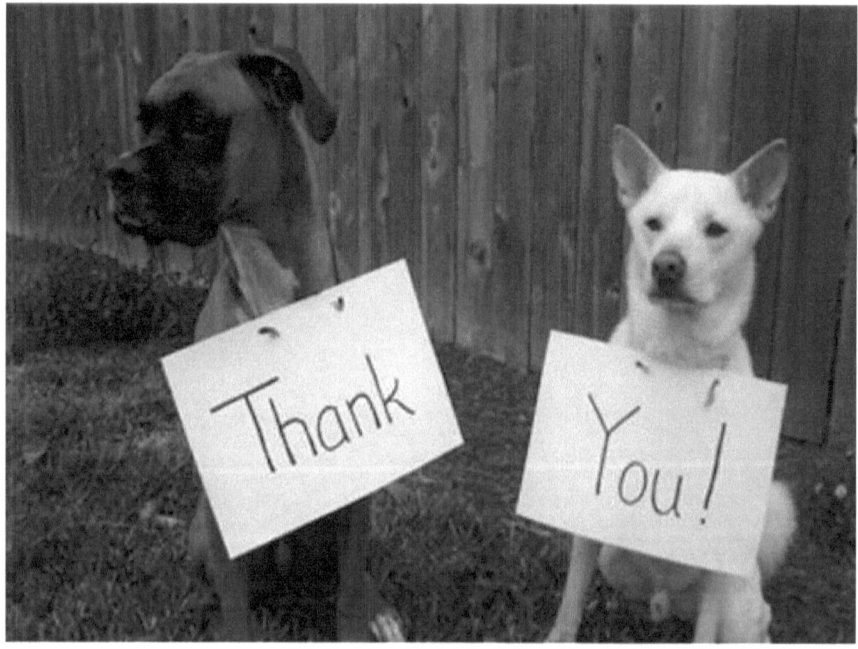

Finally, if you enjoyed this book, then I'd like to ask you for a favor, would you be kind enough to leave a review for this book on Amazon? It'd be greatly appreciated!

Thank you and good luck!